Conquering Anxiety in Children

Simple 30-Minute Fun Games and Techniques to Help Kids Take Control of Their Fears, Worries, and Confusion

information contained within this document, including, but not limited to, —errors, omissions, or inaccuracies.

Free Bonus

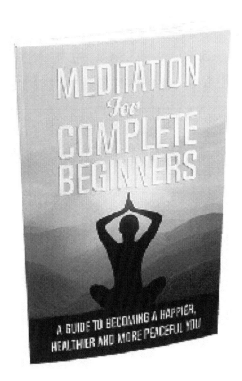

Mediation is **one of the best things you can do for mental health.**

It can be hard to know how to get start. I provided this book as a resource to help you

learn to become a happier, healthier and more **peaceful you.**

Download book at bit.ly/medicp

READ THIS BEFORE GOING ANY FURTHER

Would you like to get your next book for Free and get it before anyone else?

Join our children's book team today and receive your next (and future books) for Free signing up is easy and completely free.

Check out this page for more info.

bit.ly/booktrf

Table Of Contents

Introduction

Being a parent makes you a warrior. You try to do everything possible to keep your child happy. But what if your kid feels anxious about everything?

Whether it is going to public places or talking to people, some children don't feel comfortable. Eventually, they develop a fear of facing the world and making choices in life. The negativity surrounding them makes them more insecure about achieving anything in life. They lose track of what is around them as they are too much submerged in the sadness of their thoughts. Often, society thinks of such kids to be introvert, who do not want to indulge with others. This often results in them being judged the wrong way. In schools, other kids may consider them outcasts, which frequently results in them being bullied.

If you feel that your kid is not sharing his true feelings, and is depressed all the time, then do note that:

You are not alone.

It pains you to see your child feeling scared all the time, including in situations that are not threatening. But understand this: your child takes all these situations very seriously, which directly impacts his or her reaction to those situations.

Julia spent most of her childhood trying to suppress her feelings of anxiety. It never helped until she decided to resolve her problem for good when she passed the age of twenty-five.

Thanks to professional solutions, she was able to conquer her anxieties, but she always wishes that she could teach her own younger self about the right ways of coping with stress. Would it not have made her a much confident person from the beginning? That is where you, as a concerned parent or guardian, have to start with a kid so that he or she does not learn the troubles of anxiety in later years of his or her life.

If you can help your kid at an early age, it can save him/her from the long-term struggle. In fact, initial stages of anxieties take simple and easy efforts. But it is essential to understand that you can't create similar molds for all kinds of fears. You may have to choose the most appropriate tactics to deal with their mental troubles. It may not sound easy and, to be honest, it is not simple at all. You will have to be with them through their ups and downs, trying to learn how and what they feel about the situation they are facing in life. Children often tend to avoid discussing their issues because they want to act stronger mentally; however, that built-up strength neglects them from facing their actual troubles in life, and this is where anxiety takes its lead in ruining them even further, because they do not have anyone's support.

Remember that many kids face this problem. Moreover, parents are not even aware of what their children are going through in such situations. When you find out about their condition, you may feel that it is too late, but it is not. Anxiety is treatable, and you can help your child get over this irritating problem.

Thus, I bring to you this book so that you can understand some tried-and-tested ways and activities to deal with children who have been facing anxiety. In this eBook, I will be discussing what anxiety is, its types, ways for parents to help their children, and the reasons behind this troubling mental disorder. My objective is to give you a brief explanation about this tormenting condition that has ruined so many lives throughout the ages. In addition, most of the times the reason for ruined lives is that people were late in preventing it from taking over. You are lucky to find this book so that you can prevent your child from facing the same situation that many adults face. Moreover, it can be devastating. Without further ado, let me start by explaining to you what anxiety means.

Chapter 1: Anxiety Explained

A constant sense of fear keeps hitting a child's brain. Different brains feel threatened by different scenarios. These feelings can be an outcome of experience; a story they have heard or any other set of information their mind contains. An anxious child can turn a small thing into a feeling of distress.

Just imagine yourself seeing a tiger in front of you without any barriers. Your brain triggers signals to your body, trying to explain that there is a danger in front of you. Shaking, sweating, and other physical reactions become the product of this severe stress. A child with anxiety feels the same acute sense of danger in response to daily life scenarios. So, going to school, sitting alone, sitting in a car, or any other situation can create a sense of danger and distress, and that intense feeling becomes unavoidable after a while, thus negatively impacting the life of the child.

Not all children showcase the same pattern of anxiety. Every mind is unique and reacts differently to different conditions. However, there are a specific set of characteristics that help in the diagnosis of anxiety in kids. Generalized anxiety, phobias, panic attacks, and other types of fears have been classified to help people understand the triggers and resolve them accordingly.

Anxiety is completely treatable. But if not dealt with on time, it can lead to depression and other mental issues.

Why Kids Feel Anxious?

Generally, you can't point to one particular reason. But kids can show anxiety depending on the environment they see around them and the experiences they have. Many experts also include genetic elements as a cause in anxious children. If a child goes through a life-threatening situation or danger, it creates a space of fear in their subconscious. If that similar situation repeats itself, a child's mind can provoke anxiety again.

In some children, minor episodes can create a sense of fear too. Losing a favorite doll at the mall at an early age can cause a sense of anxiety in the kid about taking valuable stuff to the mall.

Story

Lucy, a bright and cute child, always had a generous heart. She loved playing games and reading stories. But she also had an uptight nature and felt scared of imaginary ghosts. Getting dirty or wet was the worst thing that could happen to her on a particular day. These small things became the sign for her dad. Thankfully, he was aware of the anxiety issues as he had studied them. This knowledge allowed Lucy's dad to observe her and help her out as much as possible.

It is the diversity of patterns that makes it difficult to generalize anxiety. The best way is to look at the specific issues and work to resolve them.

Common signs of anxiety

Here are the signs that can help you recognize potential chances of anxiety in your kid:

- **Worrying about everything**

Listening to your kid can help you know if your kid worries too much. If your kid gives many negative reasons not to do something, it is a sign. For instance, a kid can say no to leaving his or her toys alone. A sense of fear about losing personal belongings or feeling worried about going to a place are two of many reasons that should be taken seriously.

Kids who worry too much tend to show sensitivity towards almost all kinds of elements. Too much sensitivity explains the vulnerable nature of a child's brain. That sensitivity can lead to various physical responses such as crying and anger.

- **Feeling too scared after making tiny mistakes**

Kids do feel scared if they make mistakes. The fear of punishment can be overwhelming. However, some kids can show a pattern of excessive fear of making mistakes. Even very small mistakes can make them cry or hide. Such extreme responses to minor situations are indeed a sign that the child needs help from parents and other adults in his or her life.

- **Avoiding interactions with relatives and guests**

Shyness is a standard feature in some kids. But intense shyness shows a sign of possible anxiety in kids. As they grow, kids tend to start having conversations with people easily. If that doesn't happen, you need to take that into account. An anxious kid can avoid talking to relatives or guests that come to your home. Behaviors such as not coming into the room where strange people sit, crying when going to school, and other social encounters are concerning signals.

- **Obsessive behavior and habits**

Habits such as tapping fingers too much, washing hands obsessively, and others are signs as well. Anxious kids tend to overdo some things to satisfy their fear. A kid can feel obsessed about eating the same snack or meal every day. If they don't get it, their obsessive thoughts make them act strange, cry, or even throw stuff. These kinds of behaviors are not just the result of childhood. It is possible that your kid is feeling anxious and trying to cope with those feelings with certain obsessive habits.

- **Not sleeping properly**

Anxieties can become hard to handle for a kid at night. Not talking and staying alone allows the brain to bring back all those thoughts of worry and fear. This causes insomnia and nightmare issues in kids. If your kid complains about not getting proper sleep, it is wise to act immediately. Nightmares such as falling, or losing a parent, are also a sign that the kid is anxious. Regular fights between parents can cause such anxious nightmares too.

- **Lack of concentration**

It is common for kids not to listen to you when they are focused playing with their toys and friends. However, if your kid sits zoned out and doesn't answer you, don't take this lightly. Kids with anxiety lack concentration, as their brains keep on struggling with inner fear and worries. This lack of focus also leads to forgetting things very often and very quickly. Make sure you are vigilant about these patterns.

- **Sweating too much**

This is a physical sign that aligns with anxiety. Children with anxiety issues experience too much sweating when presented with unwanted scenarios. Even a thought can cause your kid to sweat a lot. You should see if there is any logical reason why your kid is sweating. If not, then it is possible that your kid feels scared of something.

- **Poor appetite and indigestion**

Worrying too much and feeling anxious directly impact the physical health of a child. Troubled kids tend to face difficulties with digestion. They can't eat properly and get stomachache, diarrhea, and other digestion-related issues very often. Not eating properly makes them unhealthy.

Children with anxiety can showcase one or a combination of many signs. Hence, it is essential to monitor their physical and emotional state, so that, you can act accordingly.

Chapter 2: Different Types Of Anxieties

Generalized anxiety

Your child excessively worries about family issues, grades, performance in school, sports, and his or her relationship with others. If so, he or she may have generalized anxiety disorder (GAD). Such kids put too much burden on themselves and feel like everything around them is their responsibility to fix. Attaining perfection and seeking approval of others causes too much mental stress in kids with generalized anxiety.

Symptoms of generalized anxiety in your kid

- Your child feels irritated all the time and looks stressed
- Worries too much about tests, sports, and other activities
- Stays awake and doesn't sleep properly
- Shakes in situations that are important to him or her
- Gets sick too often, especially before an important test or performance
- Complains about muscle pain very often
- Faints and feels dizzy now and then

Panic attacks

If your child loses control very often and has difficulty breathing in a moment of anxiety, then he or she may have panic disorder. An anxiety attack is an extreme stage of distress when the kid loses control over his or her actions. If this happens twice within a month, then you need to start monitoring your kid's activities.

Symptoms that present the chances of panic attacks

- Your child intensely tries to overpower you or tries to show intense anger

- Shaking and crying due to overwhelming anxiousness

- Getting too irritated if things don't go as planned

- Other physical symptoms such as too much sweating, not being able to walk, or indigestion

Separation anxiety

The fear of being separated from parents is common in young children. Kids start having this fear at the age of eighteen months. But it usually lasts till they reach three years of age. During this period, kids cry when their parents go out of the room. However, a toy or other distraction helps in saving kids from those feelings of fear.

Similarly, kids tend to cry a lot in the initial stages of going to school. They don't want to stay away from their parents and stay alone in a new place.

However, if this fear never goes away, then your kid might be suffering from separation anxiety. If it takes too long to distract your kid when a parent goes out of the room, then it can be a sign of this anxiety issue. This anxiety creates an intense sense of fear in the kid when caregivers or parents go away. Such children feel homesick too quickly, even when they are old enough to go out.

Story

For Bart's parents, sending him to the school or leaving alone in his room is almost impossible. They try different ways to create excitement about the school in the child, but he looks too scared and cries a lot. He is four years old, which doesn't make this behavior too strange. But, they have decided to communicate with a professional to discuss his symptoms.

Symptoms of separation anxiety in kids

- Your kid refuses to attend school, sleepovers, and camping events
- Asks for someone to stay in the bedroom at night
- Complains about having nightmares of losing one of the parents

- Gets too worried if you or the other parent gets even a little hurt

Selective mutism

Young children often feel shy speaking in front of people. But if this behavior starts interrupting their social interactions, then it is possible that your kid has selective mutism.

Suffering from this issue, a kid doesn't like to speak in specific scenarios. It impacts his/her capability to make friends and perform at school. Such kids tend to become motionless when asked to speak. They don't give any expression or any idea of what they are feeling. Avoiding eye contact, leaving places, and looking at the wall or ceiling are a few signs that you need to care about. Kids behave this way whenever presented with unwanted scenarios of interactions. Usually, such a kid talks fine at home or in any other familiar environment. That is why parents don't discover selective mutism easily.

Symptoms of selective mutism in a kid

- Your kid avoids eye contact when teachers or other adults try to communicate

- Chews his or her hair when speaking

- Looks in different directions to avoid looking people straight in the eye

- Talks more at home than at school or in a new place

- Teachers complain about your kid being too isolated from others

Social anxiety

Social anxiety includes feeling intensely afraid in social interaction scenarios. Kids with social anxiety find it impossible to perform activities in schools. Talking to classmates and teachers takes a massive amount of effort from such kids. This impacts attendance at school and performance. And with time, social anxiety starts restricting the child from growing socially. Maintaining relationships seems too tricky, and the kid likes to stay isolated.

Signs of social anxiety in a kid

- Your kid feels the pressure of being judged in social encounters

- You have to handle your kid's tantrums, freezing, crying, and clinging behaviors in social scenarios

- Your child acts scared about social encounters that are going to happen after a long time such as a camping plan after two months

- He or she blames others for bad social encounters

- Other symptoms such as shaky voice, blushing, nausea, and trembling

OCD or Obsessive Compulsive Disorder

OCD is a combination of obsessions and compulsions.

Obsessions include those thoughts that a child can have without any control over them. The mind starts focusing on one thing only. This thought can be as small as fear of germs on hands, or as significant as the fear of falling off the bed. Such unwanted thoughts are called obsessions. And these obsessions give rise to compulsions.

Compulsions are the results of obsessions. All those unwanted thoughts in the child's brain create fear and anxiety. So, the mind decides to build a fixed routine or ritual to ensure that unsolicited idea doesn't become true. Hence, the kid feels compelled to do the same thing again and again in a specific ritual.

Even a three-year-old kid can suffer from OCD. However, most kids show signs of OCD when they reach close to the age ten.

- Taking too many precautions from dirt, germs, and illness

- Expressing doubts too often, such as if the lights in the other room are switched off

- Showcasing delight towards routines and exact rituals every day

- Pressuring themselves to remember minor facts about unimportant things

- Giving attention to perfection, even where it is not essential

- Showing aggressive urges to be somewhere or do something

Phobias

Sometimes fear can take the wrong turn and become a phobia. Intense fear of a specific object, animals, weather conditions, and places comes under phobias. Children tend to develop phobias of dogs, heights, blood, storms, and hospitals as well. These elements trigger a severe sense of anxiety, which is why kids try everything to avoid their phobias. Clinging, tantrums, muscle pain, stomachache, and sweating are very common outcomes of mental anxiety caused by an aversion.

Symptoms of a phobia in a kid

- Showing signs of anxieties whenever exposed to a specific situation or object

- Throwing tantrums to avoid one situation again and again

- Crying if someone even mentions a specific object or situation

PTSD or Post-traumatic Stress Disorder

Children develop intense anxiety if they experience a traumatic situation. Some kids can even develop PTSD just by listening to a traumatic event. However, it doesn't happen with every child. Most children who are exposed to traumatic event feel sad, fearful, or angry. But these feelings are healed in a short time. PTSD is a severe risk for kids who have vulnerable mental states in the first place.

A child becomes emotionally numb after witnessing a traumatic situation. Losing a friend, or the death of a family member, can cause a deep imprint in the mind of the child. Without proper support, these traumatic experiences turn into PTSD. The child starts getting irritated too often, avoids talking to people, going out, or indulging in specific activities. Most kids with PTSD avoid getting close to elements associated with their traumatic experience.

Symptoms of PTSD in a kid

- Experiencing the same trauma with flashbacks, recollections, and nightmares

- Avoiding places, activities, and people that are related somehow to the trauma

- Zoning out, not sleeping properly, and acting angry all the time

- Denying any conversations regarding their traumatic event

- Being startled due to loud noises or other triggers

- Making impulsive choices and looking sad all the time

So, you know now how many types of anxiety patterns there are. That should help you diagnose your kid so that you can help your child in the right way.

Chapter 3: Generalized Anxiety

Generalized anxiety causes excessive concerns about every aspect of life. Children with this anxiety grow to live in fear of losing money, family, health, work, and other aspects of life.

Children with this anxiety feel no control over their worries. They always create worst- possible scenarios for events that are going to occur in the near future. They worry for no valid reason and tend to put their brain and body under an intense amount of pressure.

The risk of generalized anxiety is highest among children and teenagers. Plus, biological factors, life experiences, upbringing, family, and stressful scenarios also push a child towards generalized anxiety. Even a thought of waking up on time in the morning can cause worry in these children. This condition creates a perpetual cycle of fear in the brain, and the child can have absolutely no control over these thoughts. It is not that these kids don't realize their condition. They usually know that they are obsessing over unnecessary things or situations. But their ideas keep on spinning them over and over about the worst- possible scenarios.

Kids with generalized anxiety act more organized, or at least they try to. It is their way of conquering their fears. But it doesn't usually work, and kids tend to have severe physical symptoms associated with their digestion and muscles.

Story 1

Miley's parents used to think she was timid. She was always reserved, even with her friends at her preschool. However, she started making some friends with time, and her grades improved as well. Her parents were confused about her stomach pain that used to start every morning. She missed about two months of school in one year due only to stomach pain. Also, she never attended school excursions, as she complained that the driver was not trustworthy regarding his driving skills. Her parents assured her about the bus, but she always asked her father to take her and pick up from the school.

Miley often felt worried about her parents and even saw their deaths in her nightmares. This cost her many nights of not sleeping, which impacted her performance at school as well. Without any traumatic experience, both Miley and her parents never suspected any chances of anxiety. But, at the age of fifteen, her parents decided to help Miley with her issues and consult professional doctors. After a series of diagnoses, she was confirmed with generalized anxiety.

Thanks to doctors and her parents, Miley now knows what she feels and has proper support and treatment to overcome her fears.

If controlled in the initial stages, children can learn to use their anxieties in a positive direction. They perform better in their life if their brain doesn't keep punishing them with fear of daily activities.

Activities that will help your kid with generalized anxiety

- **Indulging in breathing exercise for fifteen minutes daily**

The technique of calm breathing can help an anxious child. Teaching this technique will help your kid to control his physical self with long and slow breaths. Breathing can help alleviate the mind if it is done with patience. Moreover, a child will be able to think clearly when breathing, thus making it easier to make decisions and ease out the anxiety present inside of him/her.

Technique:

Start by taking a slow breath without opening your mouth. Ask the kid to do it with you.

Hold for about one to two seconds only. Then, on three, you can slowly exhale via your mouth.

Now, wait for three seconds and repeat the same process.

It is a simple activity and takes no more than ten to fifteen minutes. Regular practice will help your child fight inner worries and stop them affecting physical and emotional health.

Tip:

It is best to explain about generalized anxiety to your kid. This way, he or she will know why you are doing this exercise with him/her. And it is also important to sit with your child and follow the whole process. Don't just tell the kid to do it; you have to support him or her by doing the exercise.

- **Make unique "coping cards" and use them every day**

You can make motivating coping cards together with the child, as you may know that anxiety leads to one talking to their self negatively. This can really traumatize children, leading to a miserable life when they are adults. Moreover, you cannot set your mind to stop thinking. This is where coping cards come into play. They can help your child feel better when he is low or depressed. These cards may seem too simple, but they really work in helping the mind divert from the negative thoughts inside.

Technique:

This method requires you to create coping statements with your child. These statements can be funny or motivating, as long as these are positive. These cards can include phrases that help the kid with his or her anxiety. Phrases such as "stomachache," "Mr. Sweaty," and "I am better than this" are excellent choices for coping cards.

Tip:

The success of these cards will depend on how involved the kid feels. If your kid is a teenager, it would be wise to give them more freedom when writing such cards. Ask what they need to listen to or read when they feel anxious. Then, ask them to write down the same thing in a card.

Remember that it should seem more like a game than a treatment. Sit with your kid and have fun coming up with creative sentences. In fact, the whole family can sit together for this fun game. Parents and kids can write cards for each other. You can also include colorful pencils, stickers, and other decorative items to make kids more engaged in the process.

Story

Coping cards have allowed Jenifer to fight her fears and anxieties. However, the technique wasn't working in the beginning. But the involvement of Jenifer's parents helped her stay persistent and find coping skills with special cards. This shows how patience and support play a big part in deciding the success rate of coping cards.

- **Ask to do one spontaneous thing every day**

Your child will love this activity for sure. Spontaneous activity, which is also called free play, is an activity where kids can do activities without anything pre-planned. This enables kids to not only cope with anxiety, but also improve their motor skills, creativity, decision-making skills, collaborative and social skills, etc. Kids with generalized anxiety try to limit themselves to specific routines. You need to break those routines from time to time in a simple manner to help them cope without worries.

Technique:

Ask your kid to do one spontaneous thing every day. Sit with your kid at the end of the day to discuss his or her experience. You can define a list of tasks to choose from. But make sure that those tasks don't become a routine for your kid.

For example, you can give the following tasks and ask the kid to do one of them spontaneously:

- Calling a friend home and letting the friend decide what to play

- Talking to one new person at the school without pre-deciding

- Sharing one fear or anxiety with a friend or parents

These kinds of tasks will give your child more confidence about spontaneity. He or she will become more inclined towards conquering the fear of uncertain things.

Tip:

Make sure that the child tries to tell the activity on his/her own. Do not force him or her to decide an activity. Let your child adapt to this event slowly. Once he/she gets used to it, then it will help the child to stop being anxious.

- **Ask to make five deliberate mistakes in homework**

The urge to get everything perfect can create obsessions. In fact, many parents force their children to perform their best in all sorts of competitive events in life. This can make the child very fearful about losing or making mistakes. This results in an increase in anxiety and other mental disorders in them; hence, you need to help your child avoid becoming over-obsessed with perfection. This small activity is a great solution to cope with the generalized anxiety of perfection, plus, it will help your child lose the pressure in his/her mind to always prove himself/herself in front of others. This activity will develop calmness in the kid's mind about the mistakes. He or she will know that errors are possible and that rectifying those mistakes is easy too.

Technique:

Ask your child to make five deliberate mistakes in his or her homework. These mistakes can be minor such as messy writing, crossing out a correct statement, or others. Sit with your kid and ask for him or her to make the errors deliberately. Then, you can resolve those mistakes together.

Tip:

Do not point out their mistakes to embarrass your child. Instead, learn to ignore them from time to time so that they can loosen up a little bit.

- **A game of saying "no"**

Generalized anxiety makes it difficult for kids to say no to people who they need approval from. As a parent, you come under that heading too. Saying "no" also enables children to become braver in life. In fact, many children prone to anxiety are not able to deny favors and orders given to them by others. This makes them captive in front of the people around him. The result is a stressful mind as the child is unable to take a stand; however, the "no" game enables a child to fight his fear and relieve himself/herself from anxiety. When he or she is able to speak up this word of denial, it boosts his or her self-esteem and enables him/her to be more confident in front of others.

Technique:

The idea is to ask something that you know your kid will not say no to. However, the rule of this game is that the person listening to the question cannot say anything but "no." If possible, you can even call other family members to participate in this game to build up his/her confidence.

Tip:

Let others know to be co-operative with the child when he or she tries to speak the word "no." This will encourage him or her to get out of the bubble of stress and anxiety.

- **Going to school a little late**

This activity will help a kid with his or her anticipatory behavior and the anxiety caused due to that. Kids often face the fear of going late to school. For instance, when a child reaches late in class, he/she may feel awkward seeing the teacher and all the kids present in class. This may make the child hesitant towards going to school in such situations.

Technique:

Ask your kid to reach school a few minutes late once a week and see what happens. When the child comes back home, you should discuss what his/her teacher said and what the kid thought would happen. It will help the child understand the difference between their extreme anxiety and real-world scenarios.

Tip:

Do request the teachers at school to ignore the coming late of your child for some time so that the child can feel more confident and relieve his/her anxiety.

Chapter 4: Anxieties In Social Scenarios

Also known as social phobia, social anxiety makes children feel anxious about judgments, evaluation, and rejection in social situations. Socially troubled children always act awkward in social situations. It happens due to their mind overly focusing on their behavior and performance. It is like having a different person in the brain telling you negative things such as "you are stupid," "you are looking awkward," or "you sound boring." Blushing, trembling, and stuttering are a few of many results that a socially anxious child faces.

Usually, such children try to stay away from social encounters. But when forced into social situations, they feel distressed due to intense fear. Many children can even showcase physical symptoms in stressful social scenarios. Fast heartbeat, sweating, nausea, and other physical symptoms can cause anxiety attacks as well.

Teenagers generally understand and recognize how unnecessary their fears are, but their mind plays with them without giving them any control over their anxieties. It directly impacts their ability to have a social life at school. Making friends seems impossible to these kids. Plus, they don't feel comfortable when teachers ask them questions. Even if they know the answer to a question, uttering words gives them an extreme level of stress. But they feel normal around their parents in the home.

Social anxiety doesn't allow kids to live their life to fullest. The fear of interaction makes them quiet, which hides their true abilities from the world. People tend to tag them as shy kids, which becomes their identity. Even the kid with anxiety starts feeling that every fear of social interaction is about his or her shyness.

It is never wise to tag a kid with a "shy" personality, especially without diagnosing your child's real problems. You need to start monitoring the extent of fear that your kid feels in social scenarios. Keep monitoring whether the behavior of your child changes whenever he or she goes out of the home to a public place. Symptoms such as clinging, tantrums, freezing, crying, and not even speaking can give you an idea of what your child is going through.

Children with social anxieties anticipate bad scenarios in their mind about every social encounter. So, if you ask them about their fears, they may give an unreasonable prediction. But it is essential to take their reasons seriously even if they sound silly, because those reasons aren't silly to them.

The best treatment to fight social anxiety is to diagnose a child and work together with your child. These kids need someone to point them in the right direction to overcome their fears. Their minds already know that they are scared; all you have to do is give them a path towards becoming brave in social scenarios. Help them understand their emotional triggers and the physical signs that occur due to those emotions. This will permit the kid to make a map of how to cope with his or her anxieties with social interactions.

Activities to help your kid with social anxieties

- **Conversation game with checker stack**

This exciting game was created by Dr. Susan White and has a high potential for resolving the hesitation that your child feels when talking to people.

To play the game, you need only two players, which is suitable in case you want to try this game alone with your kid. You will require checkers for this game. Put one checker in front and say one sentence to start a conversation. Your child has to respond to your statement, staying on the same topic. Then, he or she can put a checker on your checker.

The idea is to make a high stack of checkers without diverting from the topic of the conversation.

- **Ball of talk**

This is another exciting game if you have more than two players available. Invite friends over, and you can spend thirty minutes with your kids and their friends, teaching them the tricks of social interactions.

The rules of the game are simple. Players encircle and pass the ball with one statement. The receiver of the ball has to add something relevant to that statement when passing the ball. This is a great way to resolve social awkwardness in the kid.

- **Read one short story and discuss characters**

This activity is really simple, but effective. Give ten to fifteen minutes to read one short story. Read it with your kid, then discuss the characters. You can ask questions related to a character's emotions in different parts of the story. See how your kid understands those scenarios. And if he or she says something wrong or misjudges any emotion, tell them the right emotion behind that scenario in the story. This game is perfect for improving the kid's emotion-reading capacity.

- **Play charades**

Studies have shown that charades shift our brain functionalities to reading minds. It is a traditional activity in which one player tries to convey a "movie name" or something else without saying anything. This is a great activity to induce imagination and increase perspective evaluation capacities in kids.

- **A game of face reading**

In this game, you say one sentence and then give one facial expression without saying anything. The kid has to understand your expression and use the previous statement to decipher what you are thinking. You can give the same chance to your kid and guess his or her expressions. This regular practice will make kids more aware of how non-verbal communication works in society. Plus, they will feel more comfortable in social settings.

- **Play advocate**

This game can change the perspectives of your teenage kids about teachers and other people he or she sees in social encounters.

Ask about an awkward social encounter that happened during the child's day. Or you can create your social meetings similar to past experiences of the child. Then, ask your kid to discuss in support and against that social encounter. The kid has to talk against a person included in that social encounter and tell why a bad experience was the fault of the involved person. Then, the kid has to defend the same person.

- **Set up a lemonade stand for your child**

This popular activity not only teaches your child to socialize with other people, but also teaches business ethics. When other children approach your child at the lemonade stand to buy the drink, it will open up your child and sharpen his business and social skills.

- **Play at the playground with other kids**

This is a simple activity which will help the child to overcome the fear of meeting new children of his/her ages. Take your child to the playground so that he or she can start mingling with others. Do not worry if it does not work on the first try. Keep taking him/her regularly. When your child will see others playing in the field, it may make him/her feel an urge to join the other kids.

- **Volunteer your child for the soup kitchen**

This charitable and kind activity will help the child develop compassion towards other human beings. Sometimes people who are anxious avoid meeting others because they are not aware of how others feel or think. When you let your child visit a soup kitchen event, he or she will develop a new way of coping with his/her anxiety. Helping others is one of the best ways of developing confidence, kindness, motivation, and the eagerness to socialize.

It is a great game to help anxious social teenagers understand other people's perspectives.

How Are You Enjoying This Book So Far?

I sincerely hope your getting some great tips and exercises out of it! I can honestly say I really did enjoy putting this book together. I've had my far share of anxiety in my life and love seeing when people have breakthroughs. If you have a second I would be so grateful to hear your thoughts about the book. Hearing what my readers have to say makes putting these books together so much more rewarding and gives me drive to do more! It also helps fellow readers make informed purchasing decisions and keeps me being able to do what I enjoy. It only takes a second!

Go Here To Leave A Review On Amazon

bit.ly/caicr

Chapter 5: Conquering Worry

Parents and adults think that kids don't have to worry about anything. They are not paying the bills or cooking food. But kids can struggle with worries just like any adult. Their daily lives also present disappointments and frustrations. And continuous exposure to the same scenarios can undoubtedly lead kids to be worried all the time.

It is human nature to get worried sometimes. However, some children start worrying too much at an early age, which is not suitable for their personal growth. They can worry about school tests, grades, and making friends. Teenagers feel worried when their bodies start changing. Peer pressure and teasing also generate fear and fear in a child.

Thankfully, you are there to help your child. You can help them overcome their worries by talking to them without pushing your thoughts on to them. The idea is first to understand what they feel and why they feel that. Then, you can ask questions as a listener instead of a parent. It will make your child more comfortable discussing their real worries and stress issues.

It is essential to break the barrier between parent and kid. Share your worries or childhood problems to connect with your kid. It will show them that you have gone through similar concerns and you know how it feels. Don't use an adult's logic. Try to reach down to their age. Then you will know how significant those small concerns are for the child.

After breaking the barrier and making a connection, you can tell your child that those problems are solvable and temporary. Give them a broader perspective of life to build emotional strength in front of overwhelming situations.

Story 2

A twelve-year-old child named Mary had every possible care that a child could ask for. Her parents never tried pushing her against her will. But it was still difficult for her parents to connect with her. She didn't talk much, so her parents and teachers thought she was an introvert. With time, her introverted nature started becoming a detachment. She felt difficulty managing her classes. Her school performance was okay, but her parents were worried about her emotional growth.

Mary's parents never stopped reaching out to her. They struggled to have a breakthrough, but eventually, Mary started sharing her thoughts with them. Finally, they realized that their child was worrying more than she should about everything in her life. Her imagination was making her worried about her real life.

Thanks to the support of her parents, Mary was able to build self-esteem and recover from unnecessary worries. She still feels concerned about important things in her life. But now her approach is to talk to her parents and come up with a solution.

You can do the same with your kid as well. Just stay determined and understanding, like Mary's parents.

Activities To Help Your Kid Overcome Worry

- ## Read and write an inspiring superhero story

Kids love superheroes for their powers and actions. But every superhero character represents much more than that. Mostly, kids don't understand the hidden meaning of a superhero story. But you can help your kid understand the true meaning of a superhero.

You have to become aware of your kid's favorite superheroes. Then, find stories related to that hero to explain how they conquer fear and worries before they fight the real villain. Teach your child the values that a superhero follows when making his decisions.

Then, give a task to the child to create a new story around his or her life as a superhero. Their story will convey a lot about their inner struggles and worries.

- ## Make a collage of elements that make your kid feel calm

Every kid imagines places and things that make him or her happy. These things help them forget about their worries. But a child who worries too much can find it challenging to distract his or her mind from evil thoughts.

This game is perfect to help them find happiness. You can use old magazines or search online for places and things that make your kid happy. Give one theme for the day such as "travel wishes" or "best amusement parks." Allow your kid to make a collage of elements that make him or her happy. If possible, try fulfilling some of those things to make the kid excited.

- **Make a game of worry brain and happy brain**

Conveying your positive thoughts to kids can seem difficult sometimes. This game can help you out with that.

First, you can become the happy brain and ask your child to become the worry brain. Then ask the child to say one thing that makes him/her worry. Then you can present a contradicting positive scenario related to that worry. The idea is to provide a positive, practical thought that your child can easily understand.

Then you can switch roles. This time, become worry brain and let your kid be the happy brain. You can say one thing that makes you worried. Let the child say something positive or happy about that same thing.

For example, a worry brain can say, "I don't feel good about going to the new school." But a happy brain can reply, "I will meet new people and make new friends in the new school."

- **Jars to calm down worry**

This DIY technique is all about stress-relieving with the help of some imagination and craftwork. In this method, you need an empty transparent jar, some glitter, glitter glue, and warm water. Fill the jar with the warm water, glitter glue and the glitter particles. Close the jar tightly and mix it up well. Give it to your child or let him or her help you make one. Now, whenever there is a stressful event that causes worry in your child, let him/her shake this jar to see the beautiful glitter floating in the jar. It is a great way for relieving stress and worries by diverting the mind towards positivity.

You may not necessarily need a jar for this technique. Even small baby oil bottles, etc. can also do the trick. Additionally, you can guide your child to take long and deep breaths while watching the jar for increasing mindfulness in him/her.

• **Colors of feelings**

You will need a box of colored pencils or crayons for this. Define each color as one emotion. Then, explain to your child the emotional meaning of every color. Ask the child to draw a picture or paint with colors that express their emotions. Your child doesn't have to be great at painting. The idea of this game is to allow kids to separate themselves from their worries and concerns. You can draw a picture with a pencil for them and let the kid fill in the colors, according to his/her feelings.

• **Visualize their worries with a yarn ball**

Usually, kids can't express the true extent of their fears. This game can help you resolve that. Give them one big yarn ball. Then, ask them to cut threads describing the extent of their worry. The longer the string, the more they fear.

When you know the worries, try resolving them by asking the child about what the worry is. This method will help you learn the extent of the stress in the child. To resolve, you will need to talk to the child carefully as a friend, and not as a parent or guardian. You have to peel the layers in his/her mind to get him/her to discuss what has been bothering them. If you succeed in that, you will have a better chance of helping your child overcome his/her worries. Once, the issue has been resolved, ask him/her to cut another string for the same worry. If the string is shorter this time, then you have succeeded.

The mentioned activities are for every child to save them from worries and fears.

Chapter 6: Taking Control Of Fears

As a parent, you feel helpless if your child has an irrational fear. Darkness, strange noises, new people, water, and many other elements can cause fear in young hearts.

Without any help, your kid can hold some of those fears for the whole life. Hence, it is important to take the right steps and help them overcome their fears, no matter how irrational they sound.

The first step is to be open when discussing fears. If your child can tell you his/her fears, you can convey appropriate information related to those fears, depending on his or her age. Fear of disease, hospitals, death, and others can become less overwhelming if you talk to your kids and appropriately share information. It is essential to make the child feel comfortable when giving information.

Some irrational fears can seem funny to you. For instance, a four-year-old can feel afraid of the sound of balloons. Similar irrational fears are also a sign that your kid has a vulnerable and anxious mindset. So it is essential to understand those fears and not to make fun of the child. You should assure your kid that he/she is safe. Cuddling and hugging can help when the child is crying. However, it is also important to not let them become isolated from those fears. Work out creative and safe ways to slowly resolve the child's anxiety. Never wholly expose yourself to those fears. It should be a small step every time. Then you can reward and praise the kid to encourage them more.

Activities to help kids overcome their fears

- **Bibliotherapy**

This tested technique has been used for curing stress, worries and fears. The method involves the use of expressions to tell a story in a way so that the listener feels connected with it. This way, a child who is listening to such a story, will be able to relate his life experiences with the character in the story and try to follow a similar path of overcoming his/her fear. This makes it obvious that the story character has to be a courageous one who faces his fear and overcomes it. If this technique works, you can expect it to work for a long time for your child.

- **Playhouse patrol**

Sometimes, the best way to deal with fear is fear itself. Instead of getting your child who fears empty spaces, dark rooms, or ghosts to visit dark rooms directly, you can choose to create a plot for the child so that the scenario becomes more of a film where your child is the hero. For instance, you can turn off all the lights in your home and use flashlights to check every room and location with your child. Give a storyline to make it more fun for your child. You and your child can act as policemen and check whether the windows are locked or not. The heroic character that your child will love to play will help him get over his fears, eventually making him braver.

- **Turn stories into lessons of overcoming fear**

You have to be selective with stories and pick ones that are aligned with your child's fear. Sit and read those stories to your kid in the evening. It is important that you don't leave the child for a while after reading that story. Hence, don't choose nighttime to explain those stories. You can read stories related to events that make children afraid and how children have overcome those fears. This will help your child develop a positive instinct.

- **Play Frisbee**

Going out to play Frisbee will provide proper physical activity for your child. This will also relax a child's mind, as he or she has to focus on catching that Frisbee in that moment. The same activity also helps save kids from anxieties and fear that come to mind during bedtime. The body feels relaxed and tired from all the physical activity, so the child gets proper sleep at night.

- **Challenge a little more every day**

Choose a set of events and follow them day by day or week by week. For example, if your child fears water, you can take the kid to the pool and sit at the edge. Splash the water in the pool with your legs and ask the kid to do the same. Repeat this activity for a few days. Then you can go to the pool and ask your kid to just stand in the water near the side of the pool.

Eventually, you can get the child to swim and make him/her comfortable with water.

Apart from all these activities, it is essential to become an excellent example for your kids. Your child learns most things from you. So, if you feel scared of things and show that fear in front of the kid, he/she can hold that fear as well. You have to present a calming behavior in situations your child feels afraid. It will help your kid cope with their concerns in time.

Chapter 7: How Parents Can Help Kids With Anxieties

Spot anxiety signs

Reading the signs is an essential step in improving your kid. Not every child can directly say, "I don't feel comfortable doing that." Mostly, the signs appear in the form of moodiness, restlessness, and fractious natures. Also, you need to keep an eye on the physical symptoms such as stomach pain and headaches.

The hidden signs in your kid's behavior can tell you about anxieties. Then you can move one step closer to helping the child.

Take baby steps

Forcing your kid to directly confront their anxieties can worsen the problem. It is essential for you to divide your approach into manageable levels. Ask yourself how much exposure your child can face in one attempt. It applies to any technique or activity you choose to help your kid. Always make the child face safe when exposing them to their anxieties. It will help the child get better in coping with stresses at every step.

Ensure that your supporting techniques are enjoyable

For long-term impact, you need to have a playful approach towards the child to help him/her with anxiety. Kids, who feel scared in the dark, can get better results coping with their fear if you choose to tell happy stories at night with flashlights. Moreover, treasure hunting in your home and other fun ways are helpful in engaging kids in the things they fear. When kids perform activities of exploring, they are able to overcome their fear and become bolder at performing tasks. You should note that engaging your child in such activities for the first time would require your participation as well. Do not simply arrange the task for him or her and leave them be. You have to involve yourself with your child so that he or she can loosen up and enjoy the activity freely.

Help the child feel relaxed

Relaxation is significant to help an anxious child. Deep breathing, meditation, and other relaxation activities can help reduce the impact of anxiety. Holding their hands or hugging them can also allow them to feel protected and secure. The idea is to provide a balanced environment of safety and exposure so that the kid can fight with anxieties without losing patience.

Detect anxieties with your child

Tell your child that his/her brain is trying to protect him or her with all those anxieties. But too much focus can also lead to the exaggerations of those anxieties. Develop a pattern with your child to talk and find out all the worries and the reasons behind those anxieties.

First, ask your kid to write down a negative thought that floats in their mind often. For example, your child can write, "My friends at school don't like me at all."

After that, you can ask the child to write real-life scenarios that support that thought. Make sure that you tell your child not to put in assumptions or feelings. Only write real encounters that have allowed the kid to feel that anxiety. For example, the kid can write, "I asked Sherry to sit and have lunch with me yesterday, but she refused."

Now you can ask the child to write one favorable scenario that happened on that same day. For instance, "I spent time with Tom doing my homework yesterday."

Such exercises are highly useful when you want to shift anxieties into positive thoughts. You can even make this activity verbal and share a conversation in the similar order mentioned above.

Designate limited time to worry every day

Just telling your child to avoid anxieties won't make him/her less anxious. In the worst case, the child may start pretending to be fine in front you, when the anxiety keeps troubling him/her.

A better approach is to designate a specified period every day to worry. You can make a "**worry box**" or a worry diary for the child. Give your child freedom to write any worry he or she has in mind. For thirty minutes, the child can write and think about his or her worries, but then, put those worries in the worry box and forget about them for the day. You can ask the child to verbally say "**goodbye, anxiety**" to make it more impactful. Regularly practicing this activity can help kid give up anxieties and worries he or she has in mind.

Teach them self-compassion

The ultimate goal of every action should be to make the child self-compassionate. The pain and frustration of anxiety can vanish if your child feels compassionate towards his or her personality. Your role as a parent is significant in this aspect. The fears are the result of environmental factors and brain psychology. You can teach your child to love his or her personality and stop blaming him or herself for worries. Self-criticism is the biggest villain in the life of an anxious child. You have to help the kid overcome that and forgive to move on. Praising with statements such as, "my champ," "you are a brave boy," "you should feel proud of yourself," and others can allow your kid to love his or her personality.

Chapter 8: Obsessive Compulsive Disorder (OCD)

Obsessions combined with compulsions create critical anxiety conditions in a child's brain. OCD includes thoughts and behaviors that happen without any control. The mind of the child gets an anxious urge and tries to conquer that anxiety with repeated compulsions or routines. Feeling obsessed with clean clothes, washing hands, checking thing again and again, and other aggressive behaviors come under OCD.

Children with OCD follow a routine or repeat something to satisfy the sense of fear in their brains. This behavior impacts school and the personal life of a child.

Your child usually doesn't recognize their OCD in the initial stages. Hence, your job becomes more important to look out for their symptoms and plan a strategy.

Here are a few behaviors you should not miss:

Fixed eating rituals

Kids who have OCD tend to follow fixed routines when eating food. Arranging food in a fixed order and chewing for a set time are vital signs to follow. If the child does something unusual before every meal such as tapping his/her fork, then it is a sign too.

Avoiding decision-making

Some children can feel difficulty when it comes to selecting or making one decision. For instance, if your child freezes when you ask him to choose a pizza flavor, then it could be a sign of OCD. The same behavior is possible regarding their homework. Kids with OCD may ask you to check the same homework again and again.

Unusually introverted nature

Spending time alone doing nothing or not allowing people to enter their room. These are some strange habits that you should not miss. Kids feel embarrassed by their obsessions and try to hide their compulsions from the world. It is why their lives become secretive at a very early age.

Tantrums due to disrupted routines

Showing inflexibility regarding habits is also a sign. And if the child shows outbursts whenever a set method gets changed, it can be the OCD working.

Diagnosing the signs of OCD is just one part of the job. You have to support and help your child understand and fight against their OCD.

Activities to help your kid with OCD

- **Give a name to the child's OCD**

It is essential that the child treats OCD separately from his or her personality. For that, you can come up with a fun name such as "Mr. Bossy," "bad OCD," or any other. Give your child a chance to name his or her OCD, then talk about anxieties that "Mr. OCD" has.

- **Saying "no" to OCD three times**

Changing the rituals or routines of a child with OCD is difficult. But you can encourage your child to say "no" three times before doing something for "Mr. OCD." For example, you can ask your child to say "no" out loud when OCD tries to compel him or her to repeatedly wash hands.

When the child gets comfortable with three times, increase this number to five and so on. It will help in delaying rituals that are a result of OCD.

- **Play a game of bossing OCD**

After understanding your child's routines and compulsions, you can include them in a game. Define specific rewards such as extra play time, a favorite video game, or others for every successful attempt of bossing OCD.

- **Make cards to fight reassurance-seeking nature**

Cards that say, "Hi, I am OCD speaking" can help your kid remind that it is their OCD speaking. When they ask the same question too many times, you can ask the child to read his card.

- **The "STOP" game for unhealthy thoughts**

Some thoughts are unreasonable, so resolving them for the child might seem difficult for you. For example, a thought that not ordering food in a certain way can lead to a mom's death is unrealistic anxiety. It is vital to practice and teach your child to stay "STOP" whenever he or she has those unrealistic thoughts.

Chapter 9: Post-Traumatic Stress Disorder In Children

Children may or may not get PTSD after experiencing a traumatic incident or hearing something traumatic. Feeling traumatized is a typical stage for every person, but this feeling should heal and go away with time. If not, then it forms PTSD.

The following signs are possible if your kid has PTSD:

- Not sleeping correctly at night

- Clinginess outside of the home

- Drastic changes in eating priorities

- Nightmares about the same event again and again

- Looking zoned out too often

- Acting jumpy all the time

- Scared of potential threats

If these signs of stress last for more than a month, then you need to take some severe actions, such as home management activities, combined with professional help, and improve the condition of your child.

Here are a few tips to support your child:

- Keep reassuring the child that you are there to keep him/her safe

- Encourage all kinds of questions so that the child can come talk to you whenever in need

- Be honest when answering their critical questions about anxieties and fears

- Don't say anything that can enhance their PTSD

- Try to shift their mind towards positive scenarios

- Provide a stable and comfortable routine on a daily basis

Activities to help your child recover from PTSD

- **Teach slow-breathing exercises**

Choose a comfortable time when you can convince your child to spend five to ten minutes doing calm breathing. Go to a quiet area in your home and make sure that no one can disturb you two. Make sure that the place is cozy so that the child feels comfortable and focused. You can then explain how slow breathing can help with anxious feelings. Then, practice very slow and calming breathing. Ask the child to listen to the sound of exhaled air.

- **Teach muscle-relaxation techniques**

In the same quiet and cozy place, you can give about ten to fifteen minutes to muscle relaxation techniques with your kid. Lying down, focusing on relaxing neck muscles, hands, and stomach can help with physical symptoms such as jumpiness and sensations.

- **Make their hobbies yours**

Leaving a kid alone after a traumatic event can allow PTSD to grow stronger. The right thing to do is to indulge the child in his/her favorite activities as quickly as possible. You need to initiate those activities, as your child might deny them in the beginning. Ask the kid to spend only thirty minutes in which you can play his or her favorite game every day.

- **Design a positive mantra bracelet**

Rubber bands are perfect to write statements such as "Mom is always there for you," "I am protected," and "everything is going to be fine." You can make these bracelets with the kid and ask him/her to wear one every day. Ask them to look at those bracelets every time they recollect that traumatic event in their mind.

- **Make stress balls**

Balls made of balloon filled with rice, play dough, or flour can help child fight sensations and stress. You can make these balls with your child and ask him or her to press whenever he or she feels nervous or stressed.

Story 3

According to Hannah, it was her parents and friends who helped her cope PTSD. The professional help was useful, but she felt scared continuously due to the recollections of the event any day, any time. The parents struggled to make her feel comfortable, but time and continuous care helped her recover from her trauma.

Hannah's parents focused a lot on bringing her back to the original routine she used to follow. Her mother took her to meditation and yoga classes every day, which allowed Hannah to get better control over her physical sensations. And that led to faster recovery from mental anxieties.

Chapter 10: Lack Of Sleep

Sleep and anxiety have an interconnected relationship. It means that a lack of sleep gives you anxiety. And fear leads to lack of sleep. There are various effects of not getting proper sleep that stop you from coping with anxiety.

Stressed body

Sleep allows the body to repair itself. It is the time when your body muscles relax and lose tension. A lack of sleep keeps stressing your body day by day, which increases the physical symptoms of anxiety. The sensations, jumpiness, and physical urges get stronger and more difficult to cope with.

Stressed brain

Emotional and mental paranoia increase with sleep deprivation. The symptoms appear faster in children with existing anxiety issues. The ability to control emotions becomes reduced, and the child feels helpless in front of his or her anxiety. The logical capacity of the brain shuts down, which makes anxious feelings more intense for children.

Changed hormones

Our brain manages hormones when we sleep. These hormones impact our health and mood. For example, lack of sleep increases the release of the adrenaline hormone. This hormone raises stress levels, even when there is no stress around. Hence, the anxiety symptoms in your child grow to a great extent. Kids with increased adrenaline levels can take their anxieties very seriously and start acting drastically.

Techniques to save your child from the lack of sleep

- **Writing a journal**

Your teenage kid doesn't get sleep properly due to all those anxious thoughts and fears. Keeping your eyes closed never helps in that situation. So you have to teach and practice journal writing with your child. Ask the child to write every fearful thought if it prevents sleeping. Regular practice before going to bed at night can help improve sleep. The brain will feel calmer after writing and closing that journal.

- **Give choices for where to sleep at night**

Sometimes, the bed becomes a location of fear and anxiety for the child. Hence, you need to offer options of locations. Make a comfy place in a room with cushions and tent, offer a couch in the living room as the option, and others. Allow your kid to sleep anywhere he or she feels comfortable at night. It will help in separating the brain from the anxieties attached to the bedroom.

- **Develop a thirty-minute routine before bedtime**

Every night, just thirty minutes before bedtime, you can go for a walk with your child. You can even walk at home. Talk general stuff for about ten minutes. After that, tuck in your child in his or her bed and switch off the lights. Now, spend a little more time talking until you feel that the child is ready to sleep. The kid's voice will tell you when he or she is ready to sleep. Then, you can leave the room after saying "Good night."

Following a consistent routine every night will condition the brain to go to sleep. But this requires consistency and regularity. So you can't miss a single day.

Chapter 11: Separation Anxiety In Kids

The intense anxiety felt when being separated from caregivers or parents is something that a few children can't cope with. This condition usually occurs when leaving loved ones and going to a new place such as school or a camp. There are a few methods you can prepare your child to save from separation anxiety.

Techniques to save your child from separation anxiety

- **Practicing separation with the child**

The child needs to develop a habit that you always come back after getting separated. This is why it is important to practice separation for small time intervals. You can initiate by leaving your child with grandparents for an hour. Staying with grandparents won't bother the child much. Then, you can arrange a stay at one of your friends' homes. Decide a time depending on the child's extent of managing his or her fear. Then, gradually increase the separation duration. This way, you will eventually prepare the kid for school and other separations.

- **Role-play separation time**

You can role-play the whole time that the child spends at school. Design a thirty-minute class routine and dress your child in school uniforms. During this role-play, you have to inform the child about the expected scenarios at school. Ask them to take care of themselves like Mommy does. The idea is to make the child pretend to act as a parent when you are not around. So, doing class work, having lunch on-time, and other steps will become a planned game for the child. This surely will help in improving your child's ability to stay away from you for a while.

- **Make a calendar for countdown-to-separation**

Visualization of the separation time can also help cope with separation anxiety. You can get beautiful reusable calendar templates. These calendar templates will make the child excited about counting down to the school day or a camp. Make sure you create an excitement in child's mind when making this calendar. Ask the child to follow up every day and tell you how many days left before the school, camp, or any other separation starts.

- **Arrange a playdate with new kids**

Your child can feel relaxed at a new school if there are some familiar faces. If possible, you should try contacting parents and arranging a playdate for your child with the new kids. A few playdates will allow the child to make friends. So, when he or she actually goes to the new school, new friends will be there already. This will reduce the sense of being in new surroundings.

- **A fun shopping trip to buy school accessories**

Small trips to the shopping mall to purchase school accessories can help too. Involve your child in selecting pencils, crayons, notebooks, and other accessories. This will create an enthusiasm in the child to use that stuff. Then you can say that his or her new teacher wants to teach new tricks using colors and notebooks. It will develop a sense of fun in the mind of the child regarding school time. You can do similar things with other separations. Buying camp items together or shopping for dresses to wear in special occasions can show your kid the positive side of staying away from you.

- **Read stories of separations with a happy ending**

When a fictional character gets separated from loved ones, it hits the sense of anxiety in the child's brain. And when those characters meet again in the story, it works as a remedy for the child. Telling such kid-oriented stories from time to time can change the perspectives of the child. It will allow the child to face his or her inner fears in a safe environment and learn to understand that loved ones meet after the separation.

- **Let your child see the new place**

If possible, arrange a trial visit to the new place where the child is supposed to spend time. Taking a kid to the new school for a visit is a great idea. Show the kid every place and tell them what they will do and how much fun it will be. This will create a familiarity and allow the kid to feel more relaxed.

Chapter 12: Panic Attacks And Anxiety Attacks

A sudden sense of losing control of emotions and body, along with an intense feeling of anxiety. That is what happens during a panic attack. Not every child with anxiety issues has a panic attack, but it can occur unexpectedly. Panic attacks are also called anxiety attacks.

Story 4

Maggi always had a sparkling personality. She was just like any other fifteen-year-old, with a beautiful smile and contagious personality. Her parents had just gotten a new home, and she was happier than ever. But something changed her from the inside out!

Maggi's mom started noticing tiny changes in her nature. Looking stressed in the morning and waking up with a sad face was disturbing for her mother, as Maggi had never done this before. Also, she started missing school more often, which was also something new. Generally, Maggi loved going to school daily and only missed when she was ill.

Sensing all these changes, Maggi's mother was struggling to understand her child. Many professional doctors were consulted, but no one was able to discover what was the real issue with Maggi.

One day, Maggi came crying to her mother telling her that she wanted to cut herself. She said she wanted to end the pain, but she didn't know where it was coming from. Her mother knew right then that there was a part of Maggi that had gone to a dark place.

To bring her daughter back, Maggi's mom convinced her to write every emotion in a diary. She promised Maggi that she would do everything to find out the real problem and make it go away.

The very first page of writing explained a lot about what was going on in her mind. The sense of being trapped and in pain all the time was evident in her writing. Her mom asked herself if she or her husband had something to do with this. But that wasn't the time to lose focus. So, her mom started reading about anxiety attacks. She kept meeting with experts with Maggi and began using techniques offered. But more than everything, Maggi's mom decided to stay determined to save Maggi from her struggle.

Eventually, Maggi started expressing her emotions more and more, which allowed her to release the pain she was feeling in her mind. The panic attacks were still there, but they happened less often.

Now, Maggi is seventeen and in a much better state. Her panic attacks have stopped, but she is still working on her anxiety issues. She is thankful for the support of her parents in fighting the battle of panic attacks.

A lot of adjustments are required from the parents regarding emotional dealing. Only then can the child change his or her state of mind.

Activities to help your kid cope with panic attacks

- **Write a note, read, and tear**

Panic attacks are the result when a child keeps pushing or ignoring his/her fears and anxieties. If you know that the kid has anxieties, help the kid remove that anxiety piece by piece. Writing a note about worries can help. Ask the child to read it aloud and tear it into pieces.

- **Writing an anxiety journal**

All those negative thoughts collect in the mind of the child. How about you help the kid collect those anxieties elsewhere? Writing a journal can provide a separate place for anxieties. Then, you can discuss those worries with the kid as a problem solver. It will keep the kid from reaching the extreme extent of anxiety.

- **Putting anxieties away before bedtime**

Create a box with stickers of favorite cartoon characters. Call this box the anxiety box in which every anxiety vanishes. Sit with your child every night before bed and let him/her write anxious thoughts in a paper and put it in that box of anxiety. Then, take that box away from the kid. This will help him or her sleep better.

- **Practice coping statements for the worst moments**

When having a panic attack, many kids feel that they can't breathe and will die. This feeling makes them more afraid and empowers panic attacks. To fight this, you have to give some thought stopping terms to your kid. Practice these terms every day for fifteen minutes. Saying things like, "My panic attack can't hurt me," "this is a panic attack and it will end," and others can help when the attack happens.

- **Draw a face for panic attack**

Give your child a chance to paint, draw, or sketch his or her version of "the panic attack face." This will help in visualizing the problem and fighting back with more determination.

- **Practice a relaxation pattern**

Through dancing, you can help your child learn a pattern of relaxing muscles and breathing slowly whenever panic attack occurs. Teach them to follow a fun routine when they feel difficulty in breathing.

Chapter 13: Cognitive Behavioral Treatment (CBT) And Techniques

Cognitive Behavioral Therapy (CBT) is a collection of psychotherapy techniques that assist in identifying changing patterns in someone's thoughts and feelings, as well as behavior. This process is highly effective with children and teenagers in treating their anxiety issues.

CBT focuses on dysfunctional thoughts, emotions, and associated behaviors. The idea is first to find out what a child is feeling and what is causing that emotion. For instance, a child can feel afraid all the time due to the thought of being socially awkward. The feeling is being scared, and the idea behind it is the sense of social awkwardness. These things can turn into some behavioral signs such as spending most of the time in a room or eating food alone at school.

Anxieties occur with those distorted beliefs that kids create in their mind. CBT allows you to find out those beliefs and modify them into positive thinking. For example, one wrong test can make a child feel that he or she is foolish. Such kids tend to create worst-case scenarios for everything that happens around them.

With the correct CTB approach, you can achieve:

• Better communication channels with kids who have anxiety

• Reduction in anxious feelings

- Reduction in self-destructive habits in kids

- Improved confidence in the child

- Fears shifting into positive thoughts

CBT techniques that can help your kid

- **Providing tangible items to cope with stress**

Artistic articles have always been helpful in resolving stress issues. In kids, art can help release stress. All one has to do is shift the coping skills onto a tangible item. So, a stress ball, bottles with glitter to calm down, and other real ideas are highly effective in improving a kid's ability to fight worries. You have read already about stress balls and glitter bottles in this book. Such art objects will help the child symbolize the worries and overcome them by taking the necessary actions. You can go through the techniques discussed in previous sections and help your child treat his/her anxiety.

- **Progressive Muscle Relaxation or PMR**

This CBT technique allows kids to learn the difference between a relaxed and a stressed body. It is a practice technique that experts suggest on a regular basis. By learning muscle relaxation, kids master the technology to shift their tense body into a relaxed body when feeling anxious. In this method, guide your child to sit down, close his/her eyes, and relax the body. After the child is sitting with closed eyes, instruct him or her to breathe in and out deeply while focusing on various body parts one by one. While doing so, your child should focus on the movement of individual muscles in the body, and then loosen it as if it were not even there. This technique will require patience and proper following of instructions to work out properly.

- **Diaphragmatic breathing**

This technique helps in relaxing the mind and body through calm breathing. Experts teach kids to inhale through the nose and then exhale through the mouth. Blowing balloons is a significant activity to practice this technique. Regular practice helps in mastering the technique. Then, parents and kids make fun games around this breathing exercise. It is a great way to distract child from negative thoughts and anxious feelings.

Let your child lie on his/her back on a level surface or in bed, with the knees bowed and the head bolstered. You can utilize a pad under his/her knees to help him/her stabilize the legs. Instruct your child to place one hand on his/her upper chest and the other just beneath his/her rib cage. This will enable the child to feel his/her stomach move as you relax.

Instruct him/her to inhale gradually through his/her nose with the goal that his/her stomach moves out against his/her hand. Remember that the hand on his/her chest ought to stay as still as could be allowed.

Tell him/her to create tension in his/her stomach muscles, giving them a chance to fall internally as he/she breathes out through lips that are pursed. Do note that the hand on your child's upper chest must stay as still as could be expected under all circumstances.

- **Becoming a thought detective**

Many CBT experts use this technique with kids. It is generally difficult to directly point out emotions and thoughts that frighten a kid. So, experts create a scenario of becoming a detective in which the kid tries to find and tell clues about his anxieties. Treasure hunting and other detective games are also created around a child's fear to convey positive thoughts in his or her mind.

- **Role-play**

Kids with phobias and worries develop a strong sense of anxiety towards specific objects or people. The idea of role-play is to practice fear exposure in a safe environment. Using masks or dresses can allow a child to face and fight those fears eventually. For instance, if a kid has a phobia of lizards, touching a lizard toy or wearing a lizard can help. However, it is important to have a controlled and careful environment when applying this technique. The child shouldn't feel too frightened.

There are various other techniques in CBT to help children and teenagers with their anxiety issues. The idea is to understand their anxieties and incorporate the right technology in the right way to resolve their fears.

Chapter 14: Additional Help

Apart from the activities offered in this book, you can look for other psychological therapies. Various talking therapies are applied to treat anxiety issues in children. Look for professionals who have good reputations and respected experience in their field.

Depending on the specific anxieties of your child, a professional doctor will suggest suitable therapies or techniques. You can also join a community where parents share their experiences about resolving anxiety issues in their kids. Such communities are available online as well. But you can also enter an offline community and take your kid to connect with other kids. Meeting other parents who know how to deal with such situations can help you prepare.

Help your child understand why you are taking him or her to the doctor. Prepare them, so that, they can answer questions asked by the professional in the initial phases. Of course, doctors know how to understand kid's emotions, but your help can make things easier. So tell your child to be as open as possible about his or her school, home, and other experiences. Explain that the doctor is there to help, not to judge. All these steps will allow the child to get a certain level of comfort before going to the doctor.

Conclusion

Applying these techniques and treatments can help you hope for faster recovery. And it happens in some cases. Some kids respond quickly to these techniques for fighting anxiety. However, some kids take time and require consistent work to get better. So, you can't lose hope. Hundreds of ways and treatment techniques are out there nowadays. There is no way your child has to face those issues forever. All you have to do is keep motivating your child with your kid with positive behavior and have patience

Remember, signs of anxiety don't mean that you have been a lousy parent. Of course, an anxious child struggles with family issues. But those issues are solvable by creating a supportive environment through family, friends, and relatives. Always treat your troubled kid similar to your other kids. Don't let them feel different when you are trying to help.

Here are some final tips you should keep in mind:

- Always monitor the hidden emotions behind the statements your child makes

- Keep yourself calm if the child has an anxiety attack

- Don't punish for a mistake. Use word to motivate

- Find a balance between routine and flexibility in a child's life

- Change your expectations according to child's behavior and inform him/her about those expectations

- Always create a strategy for any changes in your child's life. Slowly let them go through transitions

I really hope you enjoyed this book and got good value from it! It honestly was a very enjoyable book to put together and I love helping people when times gets difficult. I know I relied on others a lot when I was in need of help with my anxiety. I will be forever grateful to those people I learned from. I will keep passing the knowledge along like they did for me.

If you have a second I would like to ask for a favour. Reviews are the lifeblood of my books and I would be over the top grateful to hear your thoughts about the book! This will help me in the creation of making future books and will help fellow readers make an informed purchasing decision. I love hearing what my readers have to say and it makes it so much more rewarding! I would love to hear from you! Thank you I appreciate your time and feedback! **Go Here To Leave A Review On Amazon** bit.ly/caicr

Free Bonus

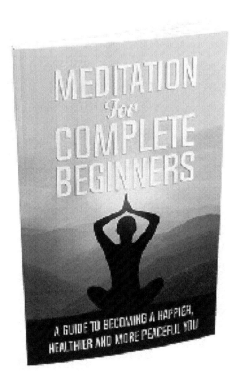

Mediation is **one of the best things you can do for mental health.**

It can be hard to know how to get start. I provided this book as a resource to help you

learn to become a happier, healthier and more **peaceful you.**

Download book at bit.ly/medicp

READ THIS BEFORE GOING ANY FURTHER

Would you like to get your next book for Free and get it before anyone else?

Join our children's book team today and receive your next (and future books) for Free signing up is easy and completely free.

Check out this page for more info.

bit.ly/booktrf

Reference

https://adaa.org/living-with-anxiety/children#

https://www.huffingtonpost.com/renee-jain/9-things-every-parent-with-an-anxious-child-should-try_b_5651006.html

https://www.psychiatry-uk.com/anxiety-explained/

https://adaa.org/living-with-anxiety/children/childhood-anxiety-disorders

http://www.heretohelp.bc.ca/factsheet/strategies-for-children-with-generalized-anxiety-disorder

https://adaa.org/understanding-anxiety/generalized-anxiety-disorder-gad#

https://adaa.org/understanding-anxiety/social-anxiety-disorder

https://www.psycom.net/social-anxiety-how-to-help-kids

https://www.parentingscience.com/social-skills-activities.html

https://kidshealth.org/en/parents/worrying.html

https://www.schoolcounselingfiles.com/activities-for-anxious-kids.html

http://living.thebump.com/activities-kids-worry-9838.html

http://www.cyh.com/HealthTopics/HealthTopicDetails.aspx?p=114&np=141&id=1612

http://micheleborba.com/10-tools-to-help-kids-manage-fear/

https://lifehacker.com/how-to-help-kids-cope-with-irrational-fears-1623455883

http://familytherapybasics.com/blog/2017/10/8/10-therapist-and-child-approved-activities-to-support-kids-with-anxiety

https://www.anxietybc.com/parenting/home-management-strategies-ocd

http://familytherapybasics.com/blog/2017/10/8/10-therapist-and-child-approved-activities-to-support-kids-with-anxiety

https://www.calmclinic.com/anxiety/causes/sleep-debt

https://www.parenting.com/gallery/how-to-deal-with-school-separation-anxiety?page=1

https://www.psycom.net/kids-coping-skills-anxiety

https://www.verywellmind.com/what-is-cognitive-behavioral-therapy-cbt-2610410

https://www.centerforibh.com/blog/childs-play-cognitive-behavioral-therapy-10-crowd/

https://healthyfamilies.beyondblue.org.au/age-13/mental-health-conditions-in-young-people/professional-support-and-treatment

Made in the USA
Middletown, DE
28 July 2021